MY WAR Mommy

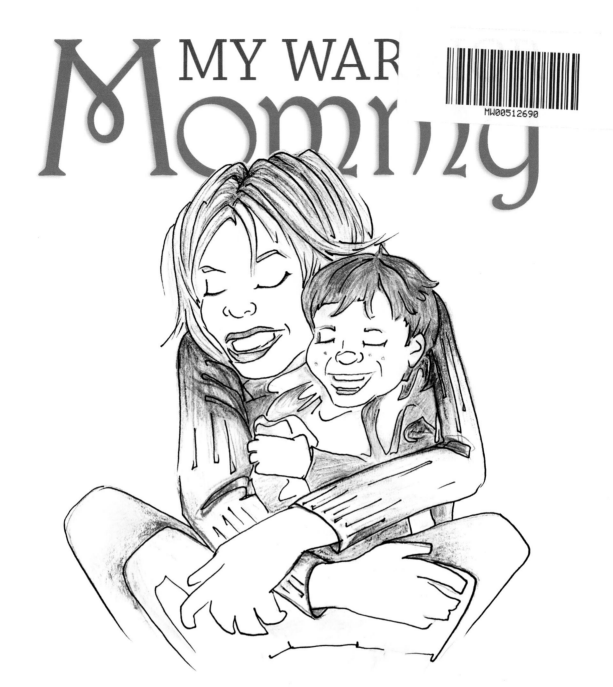

Our Breast Cancer Journey

Written by BECKIE GLADFELTER

Illustrated by SANDI FORACI

3 SONS PRESS

The illustrations are dedicated to Beckie and her boys. It takes a loving army to get through something as scary as cancer and this family did it without the guidance of a book like this one. The illustrations were designed from the story Beckie told to me, along with pictures she provided of her own family. Her vision was to show the love that surrounded her during this very trying time.

May this book and the drawings be a blessing to any child who has a parent diagnosed with breast cancer. Although the faces in this book may not look like your family, may you find strength from the smiles of these characters. I pray God gives you the clarity to see HOPE in your situation. My wish is for each child to develop an understanding of the treatment stages from diagnosis to completion with the turn of each page.

—Sandi

My Warrior Mommy: Our Breast Cancer Journey

Copyright @2016 by Beckie Gladfelter

Book design by Todd Lape / Lape Designs

Printed in the United States of America by
Phoenix Color, Hagerstown, Maryland

Library of Congress Cataloging-in-Publication Data
Gladfelter, Beckie
My warrior mommy: our breast cancer journey / by Beckie Gladfelter. – 1st edition
p. cm.
Summary: A boy explains the stages of his mother's breast cancer treatment to help the reader understand what their mother may encounter during her breast cancer treatment.
ISBN 978-1-945299-27-8 Hardback
ISBN 978-1-945299-28-5 Paperback

A heartfelt thank you to all my family, friends, and colleagues who prayed for me and supported me from the time I was diagnosed and throughout my treatment of breast cancer.

A huge thank you to my family, especially my loving, encouraging, and patient husband, Mark, who is my rock. My boys, Jack, Sean, and Luke, who are my beacons of light, hope, laughter, and love.

Thank you to my generous and supportive parents who moved in with us during chemo weeks and played games with our boys at the hospital during radiation treatments. Thank you to my dear sister for the care you gave me at the hospital. My support system, along with the grace of God, kept me in the light.

To my readers, may this book give you the words and illustrations to demystify your diagnosis for you and your children. May your support system carry you through your diagnosis and treatment of breast cancer.

To the doctors who treat us, thank you for your knowledge and continued learning of breast cancer and the vigilance you dedicate to our care. To the surgeons who cut out our cancer and give us a new look, thank you. To the nurses who administer the treatment of chemotherapy and radiation, thank you for your care and compassion. To the physical therapists who improve our circulation, thank you. To the researchers, thank you for your efforts in finding a cure!

Love and hugs,
Beckie

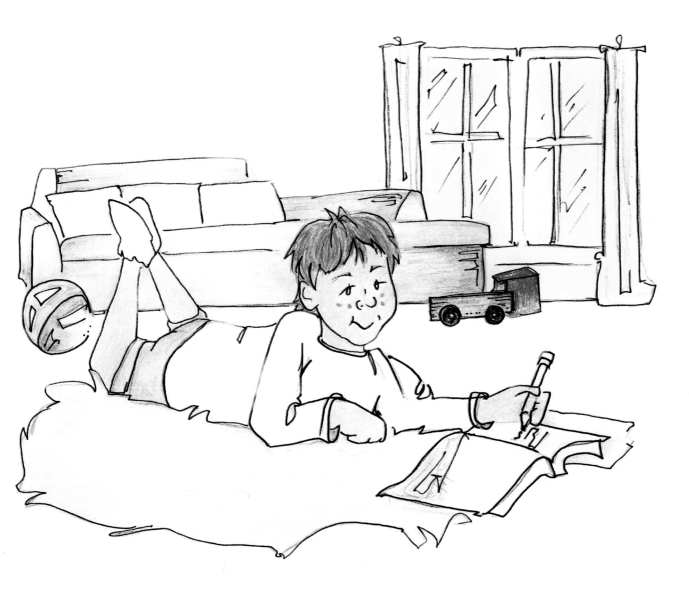

Did your mommy's puffy pillows get sick?

Did something called cancer begin to grow in her breast?

It happened to me and is happening to you.

Our mommies are strong fighters, so here is what she will do.

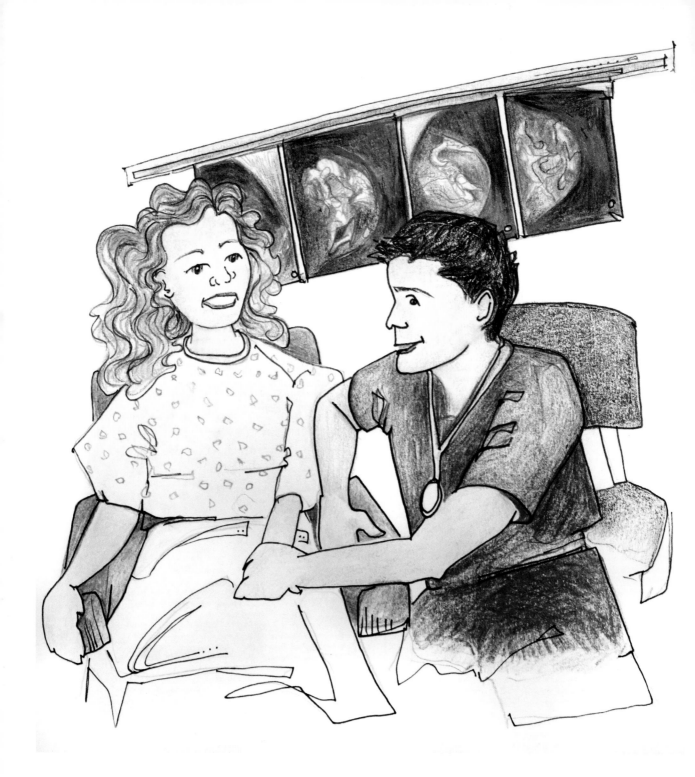

Off to the doctors mommy must go.

These bad bad cancer cells have moved in and formed a tumor.

This tumor, it cannot stay.

The doctors will work hard to try to make all her cancer go away!

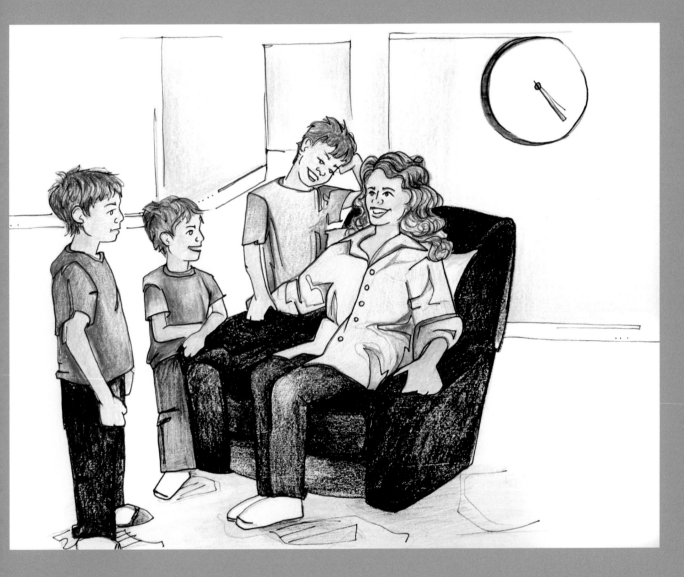

Is your mommy's surgery first?
To the hospital she must go
to have the cancer removed from her breast.
She will recover at home and need plenty of rest,
but do be careful not to bump into her chest.

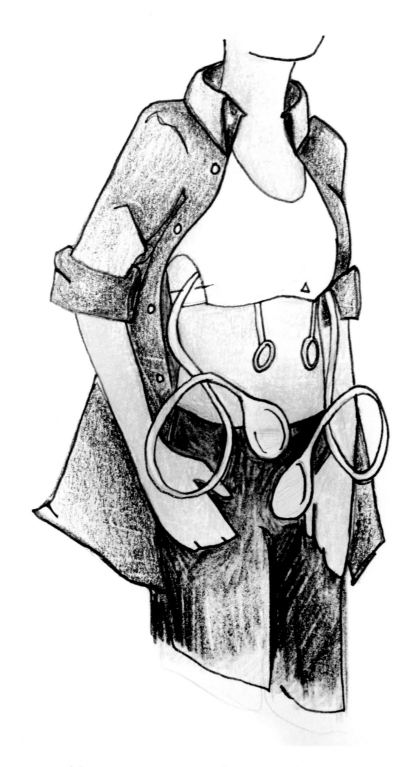

Mommy may come home with drains
and her chest will be in a little pain.
So hugs will be different.

Try a cheek hug or a pillow hug.

And remember,
This hug is a hug because it shows your love!
This hug is a hug because it wraps you with her love!

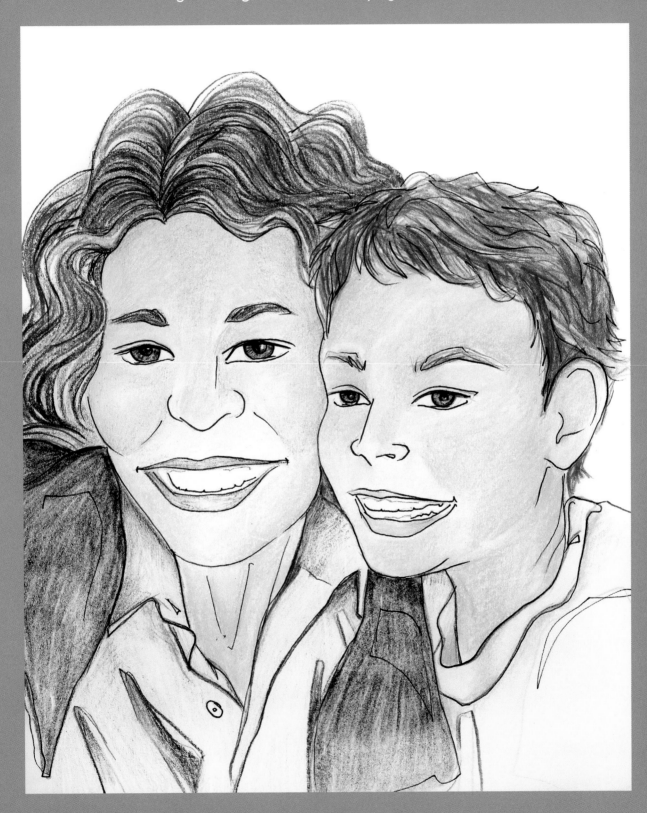

Your mommy's body is working hard
to heal from surgery and she will get tired.
Do not fret, for this is normal.
When she rests, rest with her too.
Maybe you will sleep or maybe you will read,
but next to her you will be.

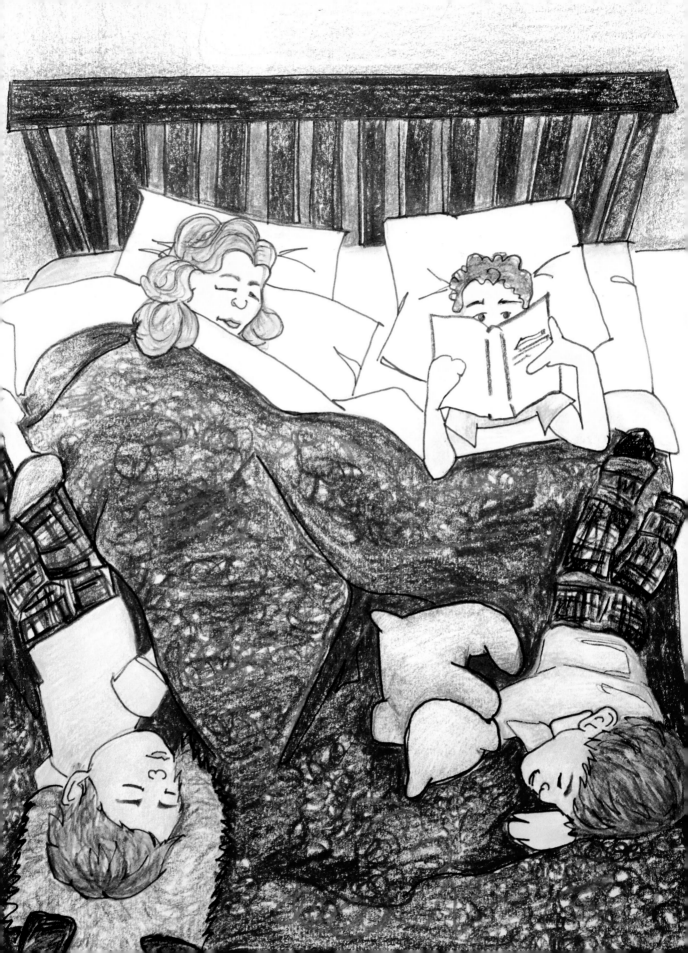

Do you see your mommy doing arm exercises?
Join her as she climbs the walls with her fingers.
Is she lifting her arms above her head?
Can you do it with her?

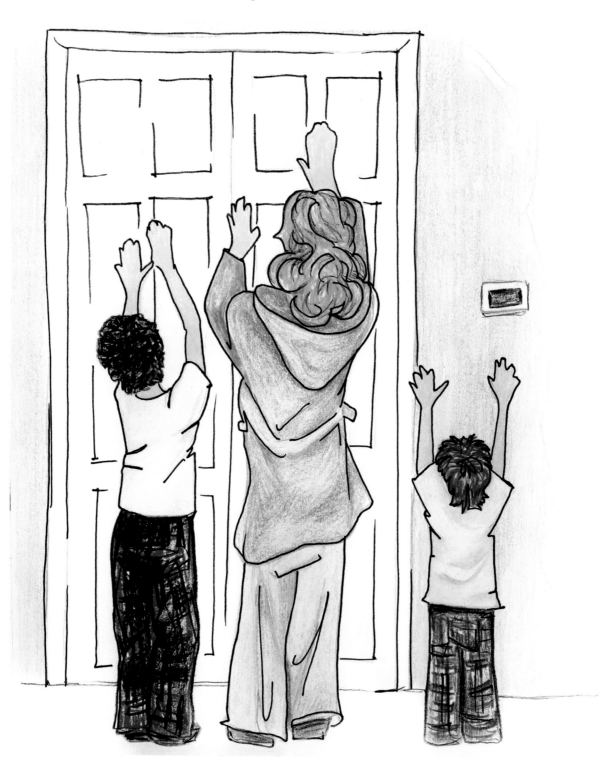

Your mommy is strengthening her arm so
she can stretch it like she did before.

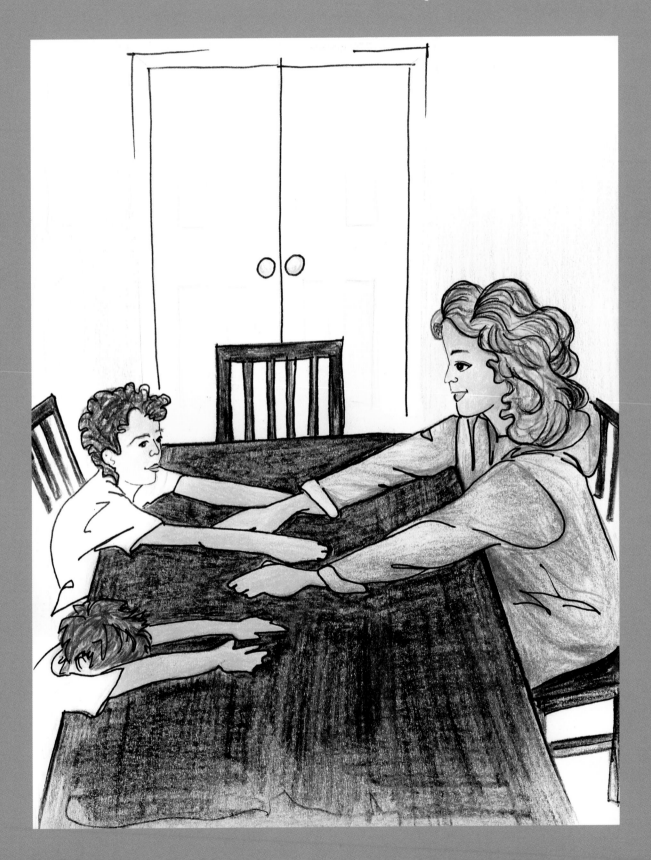

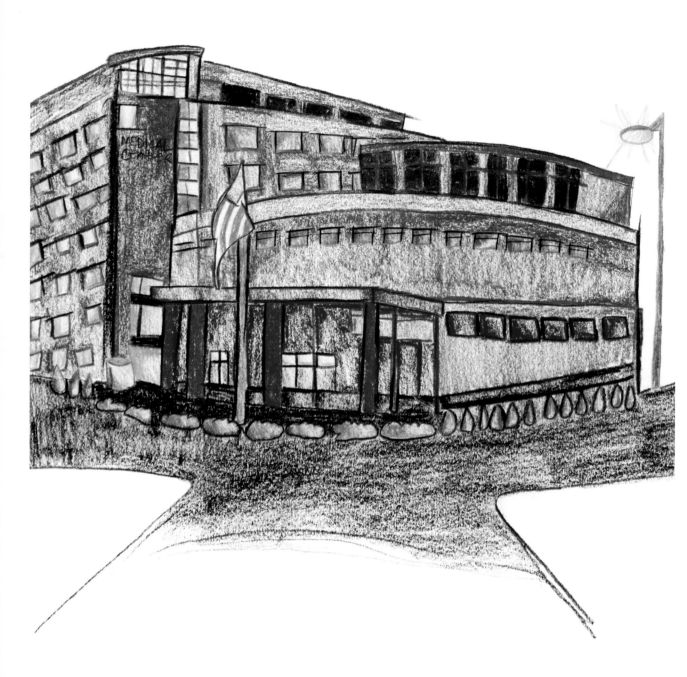

Is your mommy's chemotherapy next?
To the infusion center she must go to have any
teeny tiny cancer cells ANNIHILATED!

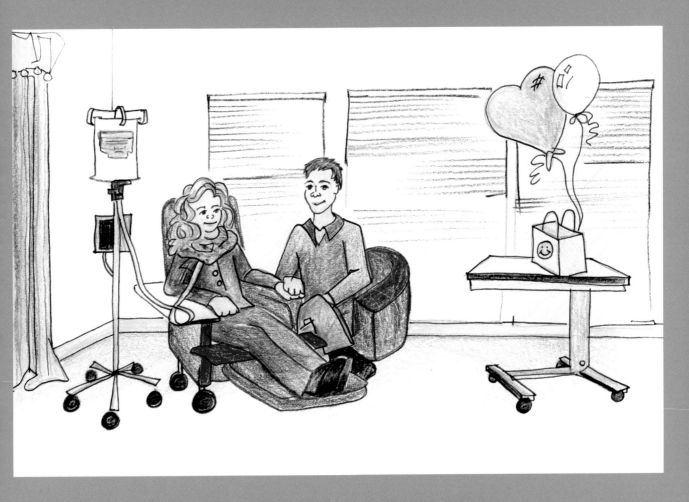

Your mommy will sit in a chair
and medicine will drip into her veins.
This may take a couple hours.
After getting the medicine,
your mommy will go home to rest.

Have you heard some people say chemo?
Chemo is short for chemotherapy,
which is like a fleet of soldiers
sailing into your mommy's body with a mission
to kill all the fast-growing cancer cells.

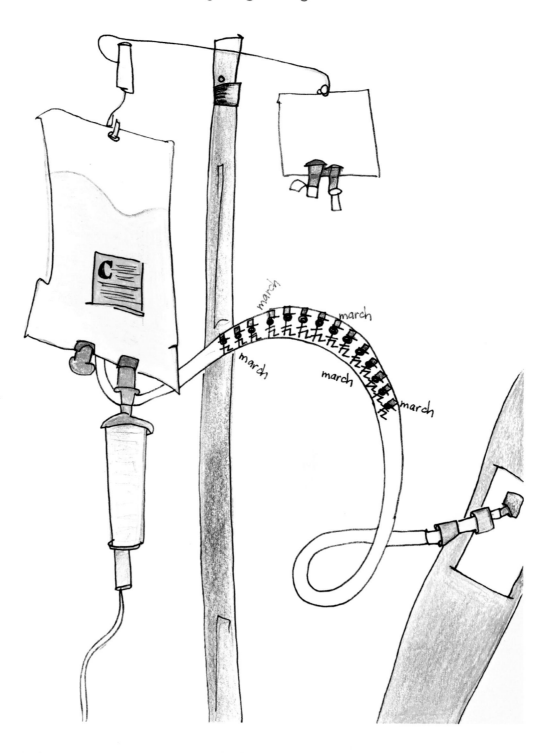

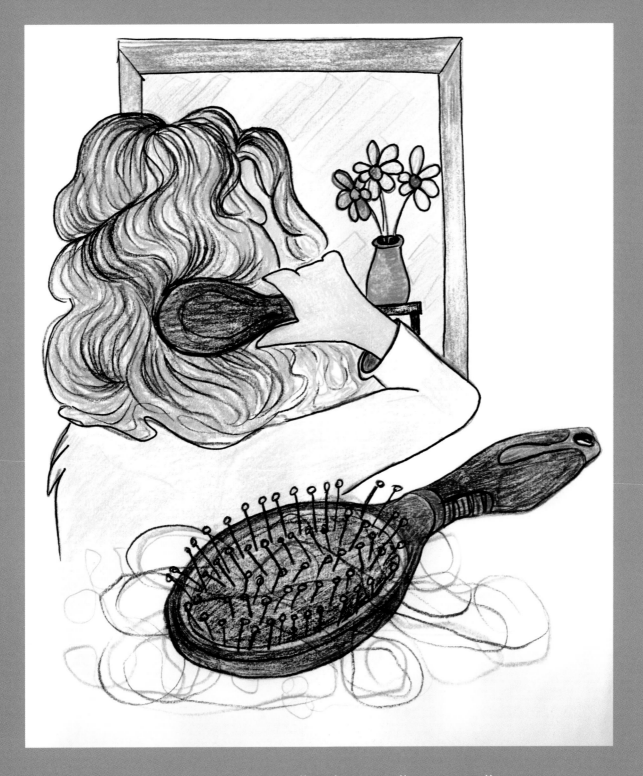

The target is the smaller than small cancer cells
that may have escaped from the tumor area
but it kills other cells along the way.
Hair hair, oh no, it will go!

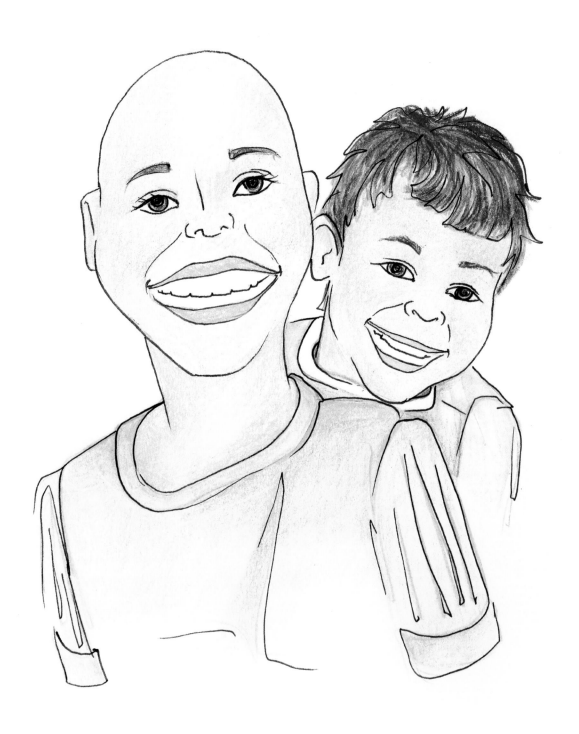

Once chemo starts, your mommy's hair will begin to fall out.
When my mommy went from having hair to a bald head
I remember thinking she looked weird because it was different.
But losing her hair is a sign the chemo medicine is working.

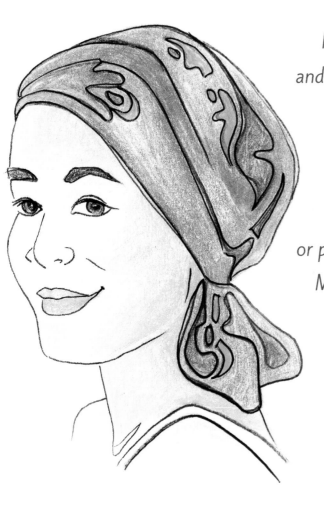

I got used to my mommy's bald head
and you will get used to your mommy's too.
Your mommy may wear
a hat
a scarf
a wig
or proudly walk around with her bald head.
Maybe you will wear her wig like I did.

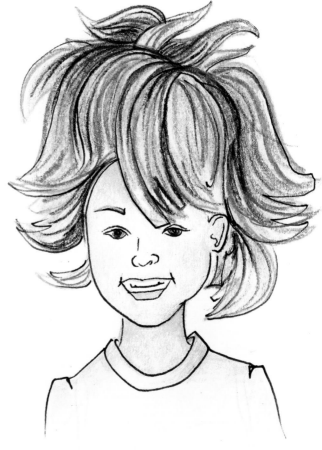

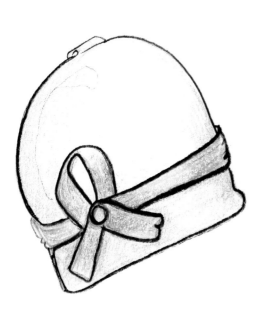

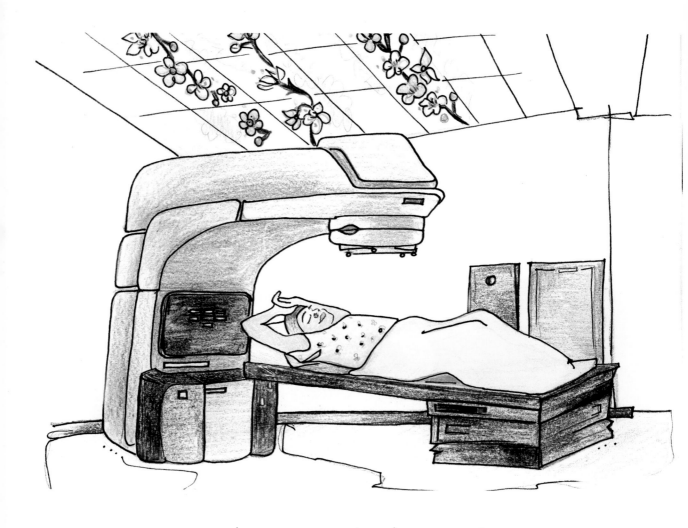

Is your mommy's radiation next?
Off to the radiation center she must go
to destroy any remaining cancer cells
that may be in her body.
Your mommy must lay perfectly still
as invisible beams sweep away rouge cancer cells.

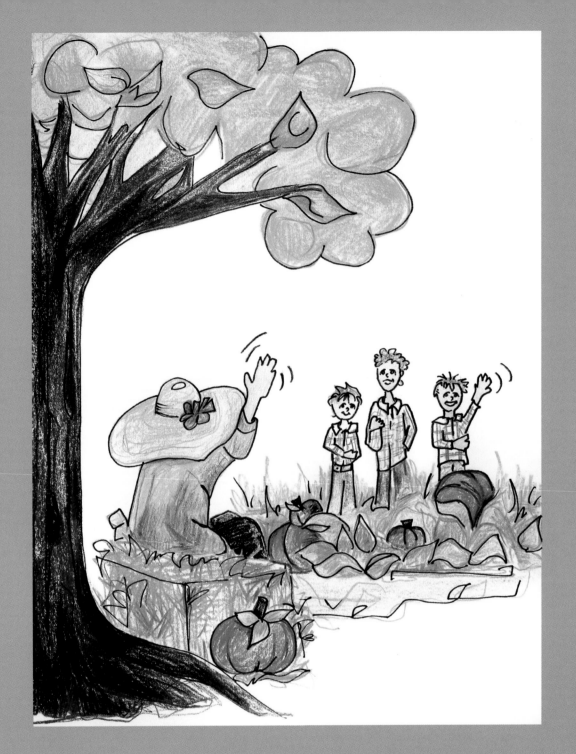

You may think your mommy got a sunburn,

but it is not from the sun.

The pinkness on her chest is from the radiation beam.

Your mommy's skin will heal,

but for now, out of the sun is where she must stay.

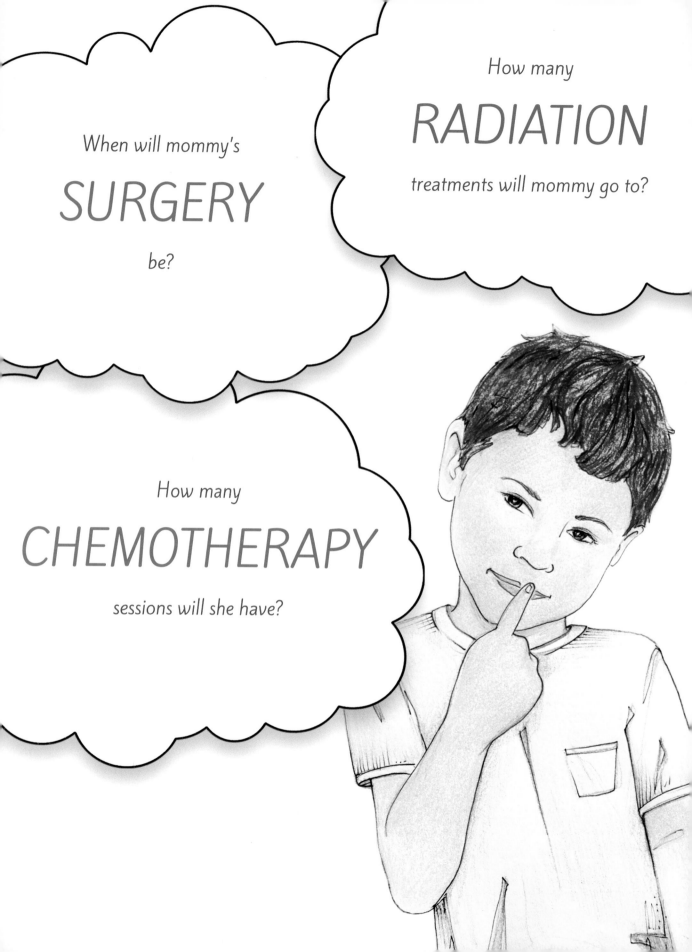

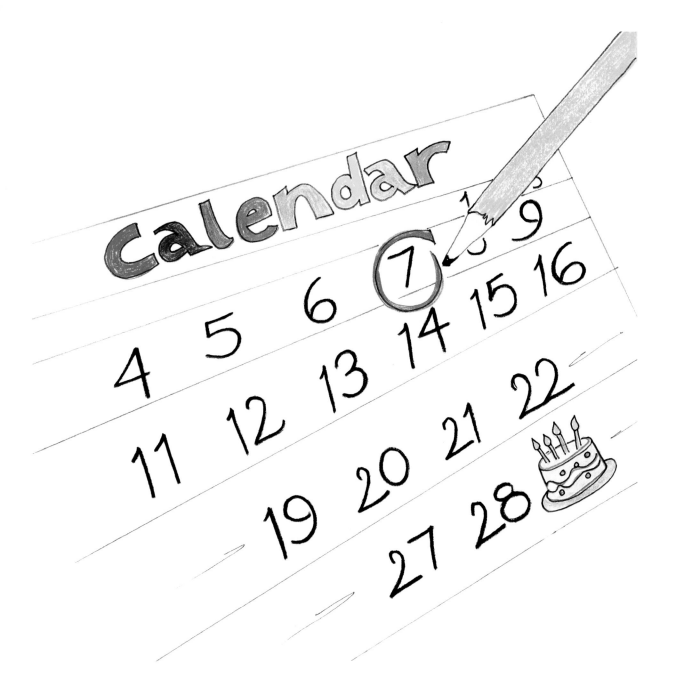

Think about all the new words
you have learned.
Like me, you will have lots of questions.
Ask them and the answers will help you
understand what is going on.
Count down and celebrate the end of each milestone.

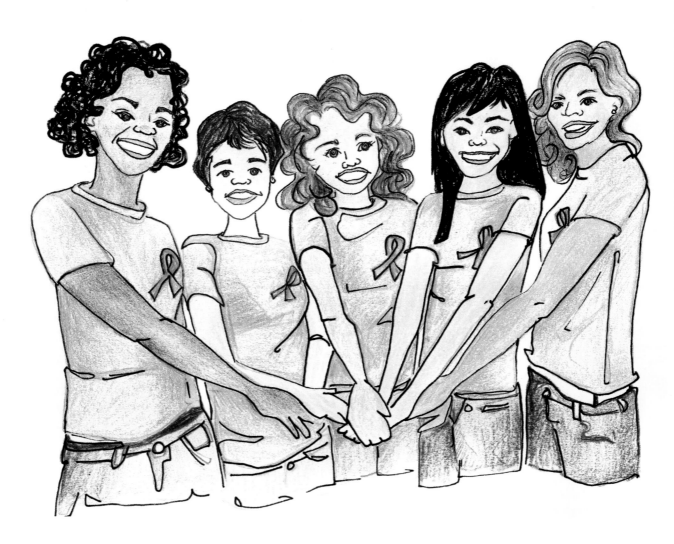

Our mommies are BRAVE.

Even the brave get scared...but they keep going.

They keep moving forward.

Your mommy is strong!

Watch how brave she is as she recovers from her surgery

and perseveres through chemotherapy and radiation.

Strong and tough —
what do these words mean?
When it comes to cancer,
strong and tough is moving forward each day
doing what you need to do
to make cancer
go and stay away!

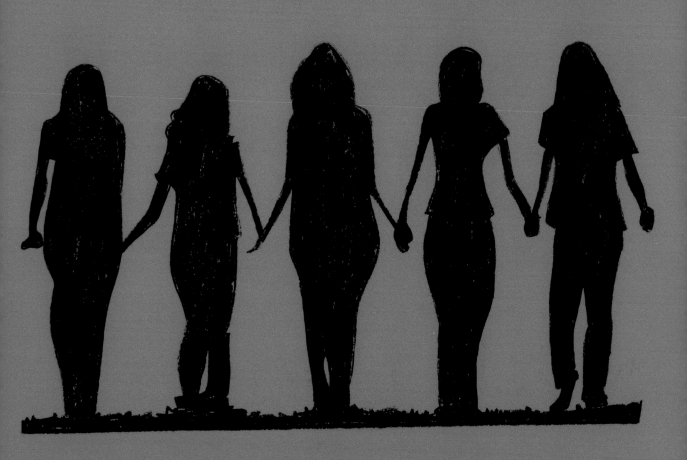

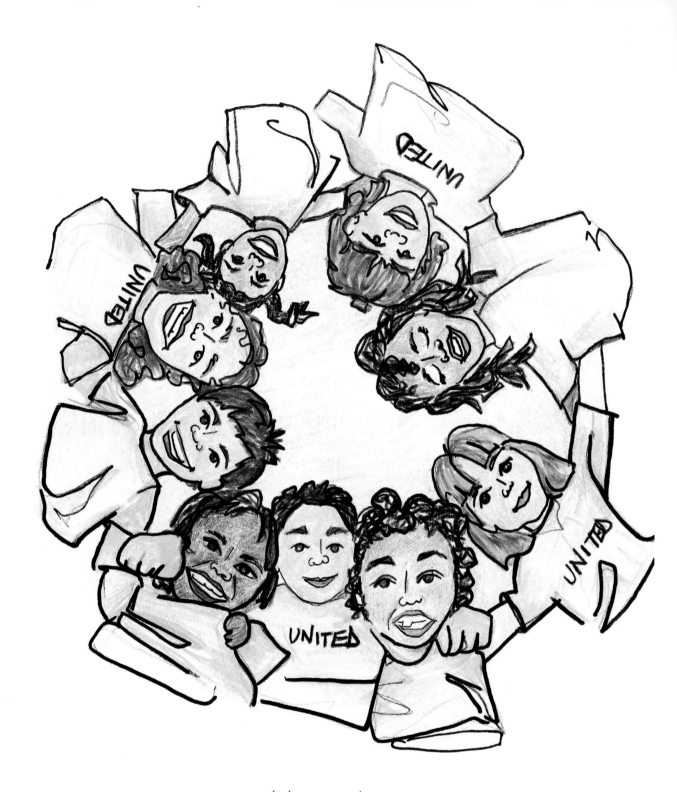

It happened to me,
and is happening to you.
Our mommies are strong fighters,
so here is what you will do.

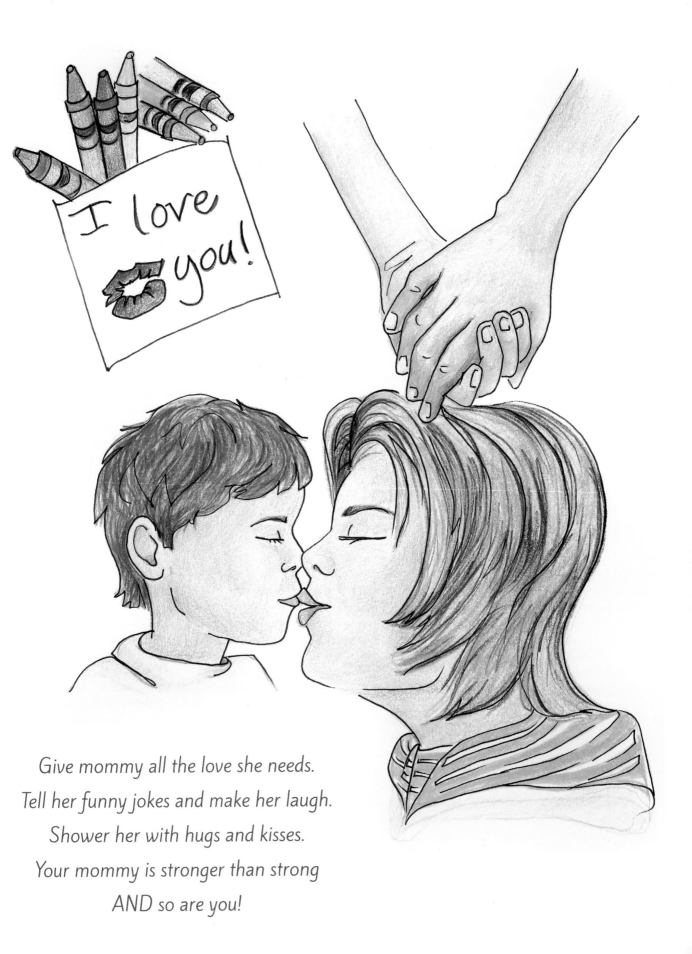

Give mommy all the love she needs.
Tell her funny jokes and make her laugh.
Shower her with hugs and kisses.
Your mommy is stronger than strong
AND so are you!

Your mommy is a superhero
and you are her strength.
Your love makes her strong.
Your activities keep her busy.
Your kindness warms her heart.

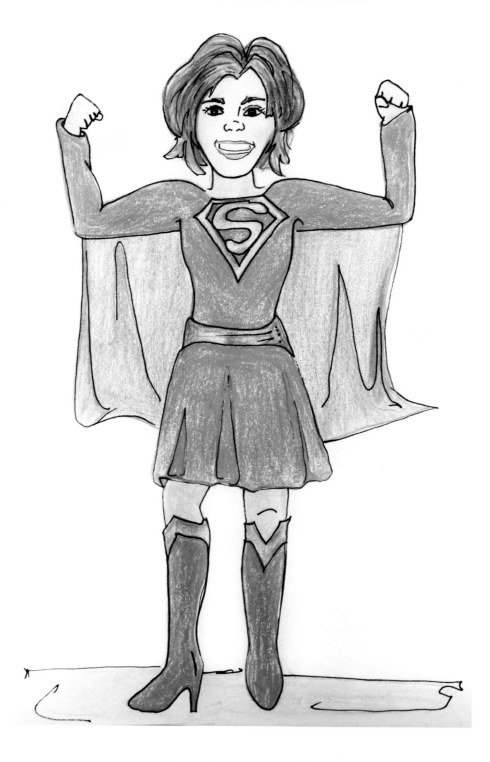

Stay strong!
Stay happy!
Stay positive!
Enjoy the sun.
And when days are hard,
do something with mommy to make the day shine!

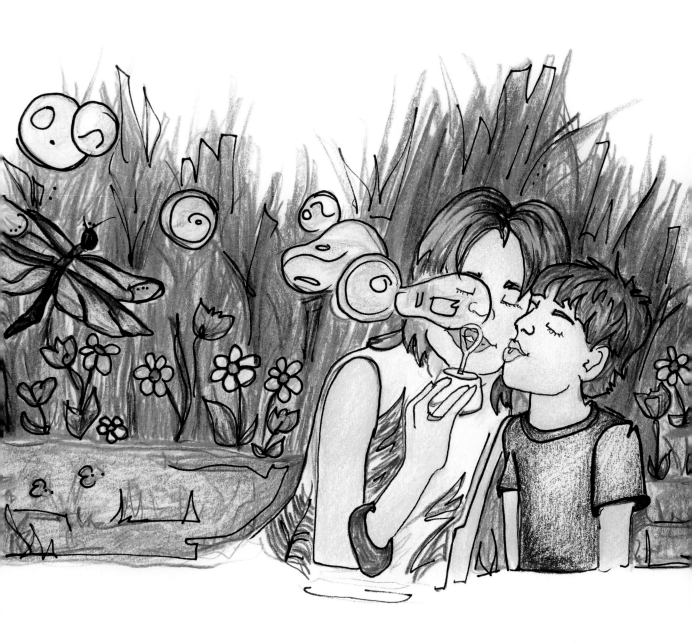

Moments with Mommy

*Fill in with pictures or drawings
from your own journey.*

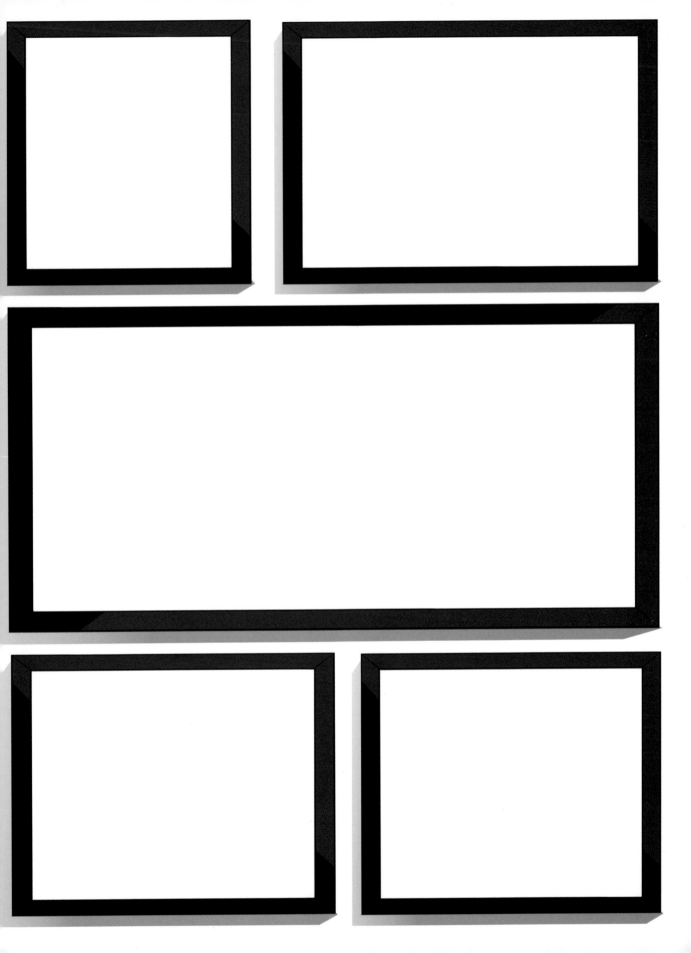

About the Author

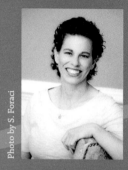

Beckie Gladfelter is a graduate from the University of Maryland College Park and began her career as an elementary educator. Currently, she is a resource teacher and provides professional development to educators while continuing to teach lessons in classrooms.

At 40, Beckie was diagnosed with infiltrating ductal carcinoma, a type of breast cancer, and required surgery, chemotherapy, and radiation. She wanted a book to help her children understand the stages of her treatment in a child-friendly manner.

My Warrior Mommy: Our Breast Cancer Journey was written throughout her treatment based on questions and conversations with her children for families who will need to explain this difficult topic to their children. Beckie is devoted to helping children, whether in the classroom through interactive strategies that encourage listening, speaking, reading, and writing or understanding a new diagnosis their mommy and family will face. This is her first book. Look for more books to come in the *My Warrior Mommy* series.

About the Illustrator

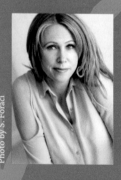

Sandi Foraci graduated from the University of Maryland College Park with an Art Education Degree. She taught studio art courses at the middle and high school and college level for six years. She began her photography business in 1998, and had the pleasure of photographing Beckie Gladfelter's wedding during her early years in business. Sandi accepted the invitation to work with Beckie again, with great pleasure, on Beckie's quest to publish a children's book on breast cancer. The illustrations in this book were drawn from photographic inspiration of Beckie and her loving family.